Meniere's Disease Book

I0775296

Top Strategies for Thriving with Meniere's Disease

BY

Howard Mills

Copyright

No part of this book should be copied, reproduced without the author's permission © 2024

TABLE OF CONTENT

INTRODUCTION

Introducing Meniere's Disease

Meniere's disease, named after the 19th-century French physician Prosper Meniere who first described it, is a complex and chronic disorder of the inner ear. It manifests as a constellation of symptoms, the most prominent being recurrent episodes of vertigo, often accompanied by fluctuating hearing loss, tinnitus, and a sensation of fullness or pressure in the affected ear. As we embark on this exploration of Meniere's disease, it is imperative to unravel the intricacies of this condition that profoundly impacts the lives of those who grapple with its unpredictable nature.

At its core, Meniere's disease involves dysfunction in the inner ear, specifically within the labyrinth—a delicate structure responsible for both hearing and balance. The exact etiology remains elusive, contributing to the challenge of diagnosis and treatment. The inner ear's fluid-filled chambers play a pivotal role, and disruptions in fluid balance are thought to trigger the debilitating symptoms that characterize Meniere's disease.

The impact extends beyond the physiological, delving into the emotional and psychological realms of those affected. The hallmark of Meniere's, vertigo, transforms daily life into a precarious dance, with the ground seemingly shifting beneath one's feet. This book seeks to be a beacon of understanding for individuals unfamiliar with Meniere's, offering insights into its origins, manifestations, and the journey individuals undertake from the onset of symptoms to diagnosis.

Beyond mere description, we will delve into the intricacies of diagnosing Meniere's, understanding the risk factors that may predispose individuals to this condition, and exploring the emotional toll it can exact. As we navigate these pages, the aim is not only to inform but to empower—equipping readers with the knowledge needed to recognize early signs, seek appropriate medical attention, and embrace strategies for prevention and management. Whether you are a newcomer seeking to shield yourself from its grasp or someone who has weathered the storm of Meniere's for years, this book aims to be a comprehensive guide, shedding light on the nuances of Meniere's disease and offering a compass for navigating its challenges.

Overview of Meniere's Disease Symptoms

Meniere's disease unfolds as a multifaceted symphony of symptoms, each note contributing to the unique challenges faced by those living with this enigmatic condition. At the forefront is vertigo, a hallmark manifestation that transforms the world into a spinning carousel. These bouts of dizziness can be intense, unpredictable, and leave individuals grappling with a sense of instability. The rollercoaster of vertigo is not merely a physical experience but an emotional and psychological one, as the ground beneath one's feet becomes an unsteady foundation.

Accompanying the dizzying episodes is the often disheartening accompaniment of hearing loss. Meniere's disease frequently inflicts sensorineural hearing loss, a condition that can fluctuate and, in some cases, become permanent. The symphony of life's sounds becomes muffled or distorted, leading to a profound impact on communication and the ability to engage with the auditory world.

Tinnitus, a persistent ringing, buzzing, or roaring in the affected ear, further adds complexity to the composition of Meniere's symptoms. This internal soundtrack can be a constant companion, a reminder of the inner ear's tumultuous dance with this disorder. The relentless noise, often described as intrusive, heightens the challenge of coping with Meniere's on a daily basis.

Ear fullness or pressure completes the quartet of Meniere's symptoms. The affected ear feels as if it's under siege, experiencing a sensation of fullness or pressure akin to the moments before a change in altitude. This symptom contributes to the overall discomfort and adds to the puzzle of Meniere's, as individuals grapple with sensations that are both internal and external.

As we journey through the intricacies of Meniere's disease, understanding these symptoms is paramount. Each symptom, a brushstroke on the canvas of this condition, demands attention, empathy, and a comprehensive approach to management. This book endeavors to unravel the complexities of these symptoms, offering insights and strategies to navigate the unpredictable terrain of Meniere's disease.

Purpose and Scope of the Book

This book is crafted with a dual purpose—to serve as an enlightening resource for those unfamiliar with Meniere's disease and as a comprehensive guide for individuals who have been grappling with its challenges.

The labyrinthine nature of Meniere's demands a nuanced exploration, and this book endeavors to illuminate its various facets, offering a beacon of understanding for both newcomers and long-time sufferers.

For those new to Meniere's, the purpose is to provide a thorough introduction to the condition. From the initial onset of symptoms to the labyrinthine journey of diagnosis, this book aims to be a reliable companion, offering insights into the causes, risk factors, and the emotional toll that accompanies Meniere's disease. It seeks to empower individuals to recognize early signs, seek timely medical attention, and implement preventive measures.

Simultaneously, for those intimately acquainted with Meniere's, the book extends its scope to become a comprehensive manual for managing the disease. Covering lifestyle modifications, dietary considerations, and an in-depth exploration of available treatments, the aim is to equip individuals with the tools needed to navigate the challenges posed by vertigo, hearing loss, tinnitus, and ear fullness.

In essence, this book aspires to be a holistic guide, bridging the gap between medical knowledge and practical strategies for living a fulfilling life with Meniere's disease. Whether as an introductory exploration or a trusted companion in the ongoing journey, its purpose is to foster empowerment, resilience, and a deeper understanding of Meniere's and its impact on individuals and their loved ones.

CHAPTER ONE

Understanding Meniere's Disease

Meniere's disease, a chronic and intricate disorder of the inner ear, presents a medical landscape where the symphony of balance and hearing transforms into a complex and often unpredictable composition. At the heart of Meniere's lies the labyrinth, a delicate structure responsible for maintaining equilibrium and processing auditory signals. To comprehend the impact of this condition, one must navigate the inner ear's uncharted territory, where subtle imbalances can lead to profound disruptions.

The precise cause of Meniere's remains elusive, contributing to the challenge of diagnosis and treatment. One prevailing theory implicates fluid imbalance within the inner ear, where changes in volume and composition disrupt the delicate environment crucial for auditory and vestibular function. This imbalance, coupled with potential vascular issues and genetic factors, initiates a cascade of symptoms that define Meniere's disease.

The labyrinthine symptoms of Meniere's include vertigo, a spinning sensation that can be incapacitating; sensorineural hearing loss, which often fluctuates and may become permanent; persistent tinnitus, a ringing or buzzing in the ear; and a sense of ear fullness or pressure. These symptoms collectively create a unique and complex clinical picture, challenging both those experiencing it and the healthcare professionals tasked with diagnosis and management.

Diagnosing Meniere's involves a meticulous exploration of medical history, physical examination, and various diagnostic tests such as audiograms and balance assessments. This multifaceted approach is crucial, given the overlapping nature of symptoms and the need for a comprehensive understanding of an individual's unique presentation.

In essence, understanding Meniere's disease requires peering into the intricate workings of the inner ear and acknowledging the interplay of factors contributing to its manifestation. As we delve into this exploration, the goal is not only to dissect the medical nuances but to foster a broader comprehension, empowering individuals to navigate the challenges presented by

Meniere's with resilience, knowledge, and a comprehensive approach to holistic well-being.

Causes and Risk Factors of Meniere's Disease

The genesis of Meniere's disease remains a captivating medical mystery, with its intricate origins rooted in the delicate structures of the inner ear. While a singular cause eludes researchers, several interconnected factors contribute to the labyrinthine symphony that characterizes Meniere's.

One significant contributor is the concept of fluid imbalance within the inner ear. Changes in the volume and composition of the fluids crucial for auditory and vestibular function can disrupt the delicate equilibrium, setting the stage for vertigo, hearing loss, tinnitus, and ear fullness—the defining quartet of Meniere's symptoms. Vascular issues, affecting blood flow to the inner ear, are also implicated, adding to the complexity of this condition.

Genetic factors play a role, as Meniere's disease often exhibits familial patterns. Individuals with a family history of the disorder may have an increased predisposition, suggesting a genetic component that contributes to its manifestation.

While these factors offer insights, the precise interplay of genetic predisposition, fluid dynamics, and vascular influences remains a subject of ongoing exploration. Understanding the causes and risk factors of Meniere's disease is crucial not only for unraveling its mysteries but for tailoring effective diagnostic and management strategies. As we navigate the enigma of Meniere's origins, the journey involves a meticulous exploration of both genetic predispositions and the intricate inner ear dynamics, striving to shed light on a condition that impacts the lives of many.

Genetic Factors in Meniere's Disease

Meniere's disease, characterized by its enigmatic combination of vertigo, hearing loss, tinnitus, and ear fullness, often reveals familial threads woven into its intricate tapestry. Genetic factors emerge as significant contributors, shedding light on the predisposition of some individuals to inherit this complex disorder.

Familial patterns play a crucial role in understanding Meniere's disease, as evidenced by the increased likelihood of its occurrence among individuals with a family history of the condition. Studies indicate a higher prevalence of Meniere's in certain families, suggesting a hereditary component that transcends generations.

While the exact genetic mechanisms underlying Meniere's remain under exploration, researchers have identified potential candidate genes that may influence susceptibility. These genes are thought to impact the regulation of fluid balance within the inner ear, a critical factor in the manifestation of Meniere's symptoms.

Recognizing the genetic threads in the tapestry of Meniere's not only provides insights into its origins but also underscores the importance of genetic counseling and screening for individuals with a family history of the disease. Unraveling the genetic factors contributing to Meniere's disease brings us one step closer to a comprehensive understanding of its roots, paving the way for personalized approaches to diagnosis, management, and potentially preventive measures for those at risk.

Inner Ear Fluid Imbalance

At the heart of Meniere's disease lies a pivotal disturbance – an imbalance in the fluids of the inner ear. This delicate and complex structure, responsible for both hearing and balance, relies on a precise equilibrium of fluids to function seamlessly. When this balance falters, it sets in motion the symphony of Meniere's symptoms, orchestrating vertigo, hearing loss, tinnitus, and ear fullness.

The inner ear comprises two main fluid-filled chambers: the cochlea, essential for hearing, and the vestibular system, integral to balance. Within these chambers, a precise volume and composition of fluids are maintained to facilitate the transmission of sound waves and the perception of spatial orientation.

In Meniere's disease, this equilibrium is disrupted. The reasons for this imbalance are multifaceted, potentially involving factors such as abnormal fluid production, impaired fluid absorption, or obstruction in fluid circulation pathways. As a result, the delicate sensory cells within the inner ear become overstimulated or deprived, triggering the perplexing array of symptoms characteristic of Meniere's.

Understanding and addressing this inner ear fluid imbalance are paramount in the quest to manage Meniere's disease. Research endeavors are ongoing to unravel the intricacies of this disruption, aiming to develop targeted interventions that restore equilibrium and bring harmony back to the inner ear. As we delve into the complexities of Meniere's, the focus on inner ear fluid dynamics is a crucial chapter in decoding the enigma of this intricate auditory and vestibular disorder.

Vascular Issues in Meniere's Disease

Meniere's disease, a symphony of auditory and vestibular disturbances, introduces yet another complex note – vascular issues. While the primary focus often centers on the inner ear's fluid dynamics, disruptions in blood flow to this delicate region can significantly contribute to the onset and progression of Meniere's symptoms.

The vascular theory posits that compromised blood circulation to the inner ear may result in ischemia, depriving the delicate structures of essential oxygen and nutrients. This ischemic insult, occurring within the labyrinthine chambers responsible for both hearing and balance, could trigger the cascade of events leading to vertigo, hearing loss, tinnitus, and ear fullness – the hallmark quartet of Meniere's symptoms.

Factors contributing to vascular issues in Meniere's include compromised blood vessel integrity, fluctuations in blood pressure, and abnormalities in microcirculation. The intricate interplay between vascular health and inner ear function underscores the importance of a holistic approach to understanding and managing Meniere's disease.

As researchers delve deeper into the circulatory connection, advancements in diagnostic tools and targeted interventions may emerge. Recognizing the role of vascular issues expands our comprehension of Meniere's, presenting an additional layer in the quest to unravel this intricate auditory and vestibular enigma.

CHAPTER TWO

Diagnosing Meniere's Disease

Diagnosing Meniere's disease is akin to unraveling a multifaceted puzzle, as its symptoms often mimic those of other inner ear disorders. A comprehensive diagnostic approach is crucial, considering the complex interplay of vertigo, hearing loss, tinnitus, and ear fullness.

Medical History: The diagnostic journey begins with a meticulous exploration of the patient's medical history. Physicians delve into the frequency, duration, and characteristics of symptoms, probing for patterns that may align with Meniere's distinctive presentation.

Physical Examination: A thorough physical examination follows, focusing on the ears, eyes, and neurological responses. This step aids in ruling out alternative causes for the symptoms and identifying any signs indicative of Meniere's disease.

Audiometric and Vestibular Tests: Audiometric tests, such as pure-tone audiometry, help assess the extent and nature of hearing loss. Vestibular tests, including electronystagmography (ENG) or videonystagmography (VNG), gauge the function of the inner ear's balance system.

Imaging Studies: In certain cases, imaging studies like magnetic resonance imaging (MRI) may be employed to exclude other potential causes, such as tumors, that can mimic Meniere's symptoms.

As Meniere's disease lacks a definitive diagnostic test, the collective insights gained from these various assessments contribute to a comprehensive diagnosis. The intricate nature of Meniere's necessitates a collaborative effort between patients and healthcare professionals, emphasizing open communication and a meticulous exploration of both symptoms and medical history.

The Crucial Role of Medical History in Diagnosing Meniere's Disease

In the complex diagnostic landscape of Meniere's disease, the importance of a thorough medical history cannot be overstated. It serves as the compass guiding healthcare professionals through the intricate labyrinth of symptoms and manifestations unique to each individual.

Symptom Patterns: The nuanced nature of Meniere's necessitates a detailed exploration of symptomatology over time. Gathering information on the frequency, duration, and intensity of vertigo episodes, coupled with the progression of hearing loss and the presence of tinnitus and ear fullness, provides valuable insights into the potential presence of Meniere's disease.

Triggers and Aggravating Factors: A comprehensive medical history delves into potential triggers or exacerbating factors. Identifying circumstances or events that precede or worsen symptoms aids in establishing patterns and understanding the individualized nature of the condition.

Past Medical Conditions: Previous illnesses, especially those impacting the ear or circulatory system, are crucial in ruling out alternative diagnoses and narrowing down the focus to Meniere's disease. Information on medications, lifestyle factors, and familial medical history further contributes to the diagnostic puzzle.

Collaborative and open communication between healthcare professionals and patients during the medical history assessment is paramount. This patient-centered approach enhances the diagnostic precision, setting the stage for a comprehensive evaluation that considers the intricate interplay of symptoms in the diagnosis and management of Meniere's disease.

The Significance of Physical Examination in Meniere's Disease Diagnosis

In the diagnostic journey of Meniere's disease, a meticulous physical examination serves as a crucial bridge between symptoms and potential underlying causes. This hands-on assessment is integral in elucidating signs that may indicate the presence of this intricate inner ear disorder.

Ear Examination: A thorough examination of the ears, including the external auditory canal and tympanic membrane, allows healthcare professionals to identify any visible abnormalities or signs of infection. This step helps rule out alternative conditions that may mimic Meniere's symptoms.

Neurological Assessment: Given the intricate connection between the inner ear and the central nervous system, a neurological examination is imperative. Evaluating reflexes, cranial nerve function, and coordination provides valuable information, helping to differentiate Meniere's from other neurological disorders.

Eye Movement Assessment: Since the inner ear plays a pivotal role in maintaining balance and coordination of eye movements, assessing eye function, particularly nystagmus (involuntary eye movements), aids in gauging the integrity of the vestibular system.

Blood Pressure Monitoring: Fluctuations in blood pressure can contribute to Meniere's symptoms. Regular monitoring during the physical examination helps identify potential vascular issues that may be exacerbating the condition.

A comprehensive physical examination, coupled with insights from the patient's medical history, forms a holistic diagnostic approach. It enhances the precision of Meniere's disease diagnosis by considering both systemic and localized factors, guiding healthcare professionals toward targeted interventions and management strategies.

Diagnostic Tests in Meniere's Disease: Decoding the Symphonic Complexity

In the pursuit of unraveling Meniere's disease, diagnostic tests stand as key orchestrators, conducting a symphony of assessments to decode the intricacies of auditory and vestibular dysfunction. Audiograms and balance tests emerge as star performers in this diagnostic ensemble, each playing a distinct role in painting a comprehensive portrait of Meniere's.

Audiograms:
Audiometric evaluations serve as a cornerstone in Meniere's diagnosis, unraveling the intricate nuances of hearing loss. Pure-tone audiometry involves presenting a range of tones to assess the patient's hearing thresholds at different frequencies. In Meniere's, sensorineural hearing loss is a hallmark, often fluctuating and impacting specific frequencies. The audiogram's graphical representation helps pinpoint the extent and nature of hearing impairment, aiding in both diagnosis and ongoing management.

Balance Tests:
Balance assessments, crucial in discerning the vestibular component of Meniere's, encompass a variety of tests

targeting the inner ear's role in spatial orientation and equilibrium. Electronystagmography (ENG) or videonystagmography (VNG) tracks eye movements to identify abnormal patterns associated with inner ear dysfunction. Posturography assesses postural stability, providing insights into balance control mechanisms.

Caloric testing involves introducing warm or cool air into the ear canal, inducing nystagmus and evaluating the vestibular response. Rotational chair testing gauges the eyes' response to head movements, aiding in pinpointing abnormalities within the vestibular system.

Together, these tests weave a diagnostic tapestry, offering a comprehensive understanding of Meniere's disease. Their significance extends beyond confirmation, guiding healthcare professionals in tailoring management strategies. Regular audiograms monitor hearing fluctuations, while balance assessments contribute to ongoing evaluations, ensuring a dynamic and responsive approach to the ever-evolving symphony of Meniere's symptoms. In this diagnostic symphony, audiograms and balance tests harmonize to empower healthcare professionals with the insights needed to navigate the complexities of Meniere's disease.

CHAPTER THREE

Living with Meniere's Disease

Living with Meniere's disease entails an intricate dance with unpredictability, resilience, and the pursuit of equilibrium. Individuals grappling with this complex disorder face a daily ebb and flow of symptoms that can significantly impact various aspects of their lives.

1. Vertigo's Unpredictable Ballet:
At the core of the Meniere's experience is the capricious nature of vertigo, where the world transforms into a spinning carousel. These unpredictable episodes can strike without warning, demanding an unwavering resilience to navigate the tumultuous seas of dizziness.

2. Hearing Loss and the Symphony of Sound:
The symphony of daily life undergoes a transformative shift for individuals contending with Meniere's-associated hearing loss. Conversations may become

muffled, the melody of music altered, and the auditory world forever changed. Coping with these alterations involves a delicate balance of acceptance and adaptive strategies.

3. Tinnitus: The Persistent Serenade:
Persistent tinnitus, the ever-present serenade within the affected ear, adds another layer to the Meniere's experience. The ringing, buzzing, or roaring sounds become constant companions, influencing both waking and sleeping hours.

4. Ear Fullness: The Lingering Presence:
The sensation of fullness or pressure in the ear becomes a lingering presence, contributing to the overall discomfort. Managing this sensation involves a blend of lifestyle modifications and coping strategies.

5. Psychological Impact and Coping Strategies:
Beyond the physical challenges, Meniere's disease can cast a shadow on mental well-being. Anxiety and stress often accompany the uncertainty of symptom onset. Engaging in stress-management techniques, seeking counseling, and connecting with support networks become crucial tools for emotional resilience.

6. Adaptive Strategies and Lifestyle Modifications:
Living with Meniere's necessitates a commitment to adaptive strategies and lifestyle modifications. From

dietary changes to vestibular rehabilitation exercises, individuals proactively engage in practices that mitigate symptoms and enhance overall well-being.

Despite the challenges, the Meniere's journey also unfolds moments of triumph and resilience. Individuals learn to listen to their bodies, cultivate patience, and embrace a holistic approach to life. Support networks, education, and a proactive mindset become pillars of strength, empowering individuals to not merely endure but to thrive amidst the ebb and flow of Meniere's disease.

Coping with the Emotional Impact of Meniere's Disease

Beyond the physical manifestations, Meniere's disease casts a profound emotional shadow, challenging individuals to navigate the inner turmoil sparked by its unpredictability. Coping with the emotional impact becomes an integral aspect of the Meniere's journey, demanding resilience, adaptability, and a holistic approach to well-being.

1. Anxiety and Uncertainty:

The unpredictability of vertigo episodes and the persistent presence of symptoms like tinnitus and hearing loss contribute to heightened levels of anxiety. Individuals find themselves on edge, anticipating the next wave of dizziness or the fluctuation of hearing abilities. This constant uncertainty can lead to emotional exhaustion and a heightened sense of vulnerability.

2. Grief and Loss:
Meniere's disease often ushers in a sense of loss – loss of control, loss of normalcy, and, for some, loss of certain life activities. Grieving these losses is a natural and essential part of the emotional process. Acceptance becomes a gradual journey, marked by acknowledgment and resilience in the face of change.

3. Social Isolation:
The impact of Meniere's on daily life can lead to social isolation as individuals navigate the challenges posed by symptoms. The fear of vertigo attacks or difficulty in hearing and understanding conversations may prompt some to withdraw from social engagements, leading to feelings of loneliness.

4. Stigma and Misunderstanding:
Misunderstandings about Meniere's disease can contribute to feelings of isolation. As the condition is invisible to the outside observer, individuals may face skepticism or lack of understanding from others.

Educating friends, family, and colleagues about Meniere's becomes not just an act of advocacy but a means of fostering empathy and support.

5. Counseling and Support Networks:
Acknowledging the emotional impact and seeking professional counseling or joining support networks are crucial steps in coping with the challenges of Meniere's. Mental health professionals can provide coping strategies, while connecting with others who share similar experiences fosters a sense of community and understanding.

6. Mind-Body Practices:
Mind-body practices such as mindfulness, meditation, and yoga offer tools for managing stress and promoting emotional well-being. These practices empower individuals to cultivate resilience, enhance emotional regulation, and find moments of calm amidst the storm.

Navigating the emotional impact of Meniere's disease is a deeply personal journey. By acknowledging and addressing these emotional dimensions, individuals can foster a sense of control, resilience, and a holistic approach to well-being that transcends the challenges posed by the condition.

Strategies for Dealing with Anxiety and Stress in Meniere's Disease

Meniere's disease, with its unpredictable nature and challenging symptoms, often brings a heightened sense of anxiety and stress. Managing these emotional responses becomes a crucial component of the journey, empowering individuals to navigate the storm with resilience and a sense of control.

1. Education and Understanding:

Knowledge is a powerful antidote to anxiety. Understanding the mechanics of Meniere's disease, its triggers, and the nature of symptoms can demystify the condition. Educational resources, discussions with healthcare professionals, and participation in support groups contribute to a sense of empowerment and control over the unknown.

2. Mindfulness and Relaxation Techniques:

Mindfulness and relaxation techniques serve as anchors in the tumult of anxiety. Practices such as deep breathing, progressive muscle relaxation, and guided imagery provide tools for calming the nervous system, promoting a sense of tranquility amidst the chaos.

3. Cognitive Behavioral Therapy (CBT):
CBT, a therapeutic approach, helps individuals identify and modify negative thought patterns. By addressing anxious thoughts and developing healthier coping mechanisms, CBT becomes a valuable tool in managing the mental and emotional impact of Meniere's.

4. Stress Management Strategies:
Proactive stress management is essential in the Meniere's journey. Incorporating stress-reducing practices into daily life, such as regular exercise, adequate sleep, and engaging in enjoyable activities, forms a protective shield against the exacerbation of symptoms triggered by stress.

5. Communication and Support Systems:
Open communication with loved ones, friends, and colleagues about the challenges posed by Meniere's fosters understanding and support. Establishing a robust support system creates a network of individuals who can offer assistance during moments of heightened stress.

6. Professional Counseling:
For those facing persistent anxiety or overwhelming stress, seeking professional counseling becomes a valuable step. Mental health professionals provide tailored strategies and a safe space for individuals to explore and address the emotional impact of Meniere's disease.

7. Adaptive Coping Strategies:
Developing adaptive coping strategies is an ongoing process. These strategies may include establishing a routine, setting realistic goals, and employing effective time management techniques to mitigate stressors and foster a sense of stability.

In the complex landscape of Meniere's disease, managing anxiety and stress is not a one-size-fits-all endeavor. It involves a personalized and dynamic approach, blending various strategies to create a toolkit for emotional well-being. By proactively addressing anxiety and stress, individuals can cultivate resilience and enhance their ability to weather the challenges inherent in living with Meniere's disease.

The Crucial Role of Support Groups and Counseling in Meniere's Journey

Meniere's disease, with its labyrinthine challenges, extends beyond the physical realm, impacting the emotional and mental well-being of those navigating its unpredictable course. In this intricate landscape, support groups and counseling emerge as beacons of understanding, empathy, and resilience, offering individuals a lifeline as they traverse the complex emotional terrain of Meniere's.

1. Shared Understanding and Empathy:
Participating in support groups provides a unique space where individuals can share their experiences, fears, and triumphs with others who intimately understand the nuances of living with Meniere's. The shared understanding within these groups fosters empathy, reducing feelings of isolation and offering a sense of validation to individual struggles.

2. Learning Coping Strategies:
Support groups become invaluable arenas for learning and sharing coping strategies. Practical tips for managing symptoms, navigating healthcare systems, and coping with the emotional impact of Meniere's are exchanged. This collective wisdom empowers individuals with a diverse toolkit to enhance their resilience and adaptability.

3. Validation of Emotional Struggles:
Counseling, whether individual or group-based, offers a confidential and supportive space for individuals to explore and navigate the emotional challenges of Meniere's disease. Validation of these struggles by a trained mental health professional normalizes the emotional response to a chronic condition, reducing the stigma often associated with mental health.

4. Strategic Coping Skills:
Counseling equips individuals with strategic coping skills tailored to their unique emotional landscape. Cognitive-behavioral techniques, stress management strategies, and goal-setting exercises become powerful tools in managing anxiety, stress, and depressive symptoms.

5. Enhanced Emotional Resilience:
Participation in support groups and counseling contributes to the development of enhanced emotional resilience. Individuals learn to navigate the ebb and flow of Meniere's symptoms with a sense of agency, embracing the emotional facets of their journey with a proactive mindset.

6. Educational Opportunities:
Beyond emotional support, support groups often provide educational opportunities, featuring guest speakers, workshops, and resources that empower individuals with knowledge about Meniere's disease. Informed individuals are better equipped to make decisions about their healthcare and well-being.

In the intricate tapestry of Meniere's, where the physical, emotional, and mental aspects intertwine, the importance of support groups and counseling becomes undeniable. These avenues of support offer solace, understanding, and practical tools for individuals to navigate the challenges of Meniere's with resilience, grace, and a sense of shared humanity.

CHAPTER FOUR

Harmony in Lifestyle

Living with Meniere's disease often prompts a symphony of lifestyle modifications, each note harmonizing to create an environment conducive to well-being. These adjustments, both practical and holistic, empower individuals to navigate the challenges presented by vertigo, hearing loss, tinnitus, and ear fullness.

1. Dietary Changes:
Exploring dietary modifications stands out as a significant step in managing Meniere's. Individuals often find relief by reducing sodium intake, as excess salt can contribute to fluid retention in the inner ear, exacerbating symptoms. Additionally, some individuals find benefits in avoiding specific trigger foods such as caffeine, alcohol, and processed sugars.

2. Hydration Habits:

Maintaining optimal hydration is crucial for individuals with Meniere's disease. Proper fluid balance in the body can contribute to a stable environment within the inner ear. Consistent and adequate water intake is a simple yet effective lifestyle modification.

3. Stress Management:
Given the intricate connection between stress and Meniere's symptoms, adopting stress management techniques is paramount. Practices such as meditation, yoga, and mindfulness not only enhance emotional well-being but also contribute to symptom mitigation by promoting overall relaxation.

4. Regular Exercise:
Engaging in regular exercise is a lifestyle modification with multifaceted benefits. Physical activity supports cardiovascular health, helps manage stress, and contributes to overall well-being. Tailoring exercise routines to individual abilities and preferences is essential in fostering consistency.

5. Sleep Hygiene:
Prioritizing good sleep hygiene is crucial for individuals with Meniere's. Establishing a consistent sleep schedule, creating a conducive sleep environment, and incorporating relaxation techniques before bedtime contribute to quality rest, which is vital for overall health and symptom management.

6. Vestibular Rehabilitation:

Incorporating vestibular rehabilitation exercises into daily routines is a targeted lifestyle modification. These exercises aim to improve balance and coordination, addressing the vestibular component of Meniere's disease. Guidance from a healthcare professional ensures these exercises are tailored to individual needs and capabilities.

7. Environmental Adaptations:

Adapting the immediate environment is another facet of lifestyle modification. Minimizing potential hazards in the living space, considering ergonomic adjustments, and employing supportive devices contribute to creating a safe and comfortable atmosphere.

8. Holistic Well-Being:

Embracing holistic well-being involves considering the interconnected aspects of physical, emotional, and mental health. Engaging in activities that bring joy, connecting with supportive communities, and nurturing relationships contribute to a comprehensive approach to living with Meniere's.

Lifestyle modifications in the Meniere's journey are not rigid rules but personalized adjustments that empower individuals to reclaim agency over their well-being. By fostering a proactive and adaptive mindset, individuals can craft a lifestyle that not only mitigates symptoms but enhances their overall quality of life amidst the challenges posed by Meniere's disease.

Stress Management Techniques for Meniere's Warriors

Navigating the unpredictable seas of Meniere's disease often brings waves of stress and anxiety. Crafting an arsenal of stress management techniques becomes essential for individuals seeking to find harmony amidst the turbulence of symptoms.

1. Mindfulness Meditation:
Mindfulness meditation cultivates present-moment awareness, providing a refuge from the whirlwind of thoughts. Focusing on the breath and grounding oneself in the now helps alleviate stress and promote a sense of calm.

2. Deep Breathing Exercises:
Simple yet potent, deep breathing exercises reduce physiological stress responses. Techniques like diaphragmatic breathing or box breathing, where inhalation and exhalation are consciously extended, enhance relaxation and support emotional well-being.

3. Progressive Muscle Relaxation (PMR):

Progressive Muscle Relaxation involves systematically tensing and relaxing muscle groups, releasing physical tension. This systematic approach not only eases muscular stress but also contributes to overall relaxation.

4. Yoga and Tai Chi:

Yoga and Tai Chi blend movement with mindfulness, promoting flexibility, balance, and mental calmness. These practices, adaptable to various fitness levels, offer holistic benefits for stress reduction.

5. Guided Imagery:

Guided imagery involves creating a mental image of a peaceful, serene place, fostering relaxation. Visualization of tranquil scenes, guided by calming narration or personal imagination, serves as a powerful tool in stress management.

6. Regular Exercise:

Physical activity is a natural stress buster, releasing endorphins that uplift mood. Tailoring exercise routines to individual preferences and capabilities ensures consistency and maximizes stress-relieving benefits.

7. Time Management:

Efficient time management minimizes stress triggers. Prioritizing tasks, breaking them into manageable steps, and incorporating breaks contribute to a sense of control over daily demands.

Embracing these stress management techniques empowers individuals with Meniere's disease to navigate the challenges with resilience. By weaving these practices into daily life, individuals not only alleviate stress but foster a proactive and adaptive mindset, creating a harmonious melody amidst the uncertainties of living with Meniere's.

Balance Strategies and Exercises for Meniere's Disease

Meniere's disease, with its disruptive impact on the vestibular system, underscores the importance of adopting balance strategies and exercises to enhance stability and reduce the risk of falls. These targeted interventions contribute to the overall management of Meniere's symptoms and improve the quality of life for those grappling with this intricate condition.

1. Vestibular Rehabilitation Exercises:
Vestibular rehabilitation exercises are tailored exercises designed to improve balance and coordination. These exercises, prescribed by healthcare professionals, target the vestibular system, helping individuals adapt to

changes in their sense of balance and reduce the severity and frequency of vertigo episodes.

2. Tai Chi:
The ancient practice of Tai Chi combines slow, flowing movements with mindfulness, promoting balance, flexibility, and coordination. Incorporating Tai Chi into a routine provides both physical and mental benefits, fostering a sense of equilibrium in individuals with Meniere's.

3. Balance Training:
Balance training involves specific exercises that challenge and improve stability. Simple activities like standing on one leg or walking heel-to-toe can be incorporated into daily routines, gradually enhancing balance over time.

4. Yoga:
Yoga, with its emphasis on body awareness and controlled movements, aids in balance improvement. Modified poses and sequences can be adapted to individual abilities, offering a gentle yet effective way to enhance stability.

5. Head and Eye Movement Exercises:
Exercises that involve controlled head and eye movements contribute to vestibular adaptation. These exercises mimic the motions that may trigger vertigo,

helping the vestibular system adjust and reducing sensitivity to certain movements.

6. Adaptations to Environment:
Making environmental adaptations is a practical strategy to prevent falls. Ensuring proper lighting, removing tripping hazards, and using supportive aids like handrails can create a safer living space for individuals with Meniere's.

Incorporating these balance strategies and exercises into daily life not only enhances physical stability but also instills confidence in individuals navigating the challenges of Meniere's disease. The proactive approach to balance maintenance contributes to an improved sense of well-being and empowers individuals to face the dynamic nature of their condition with resilience.

The Crucial Role of Regular Exercise in Meniere's Management

In the intricate journey of Meniere's disease, regular exercise emerges as a powerful ally in promoting overall well-being and mitigating the impact of its complex symptoms. Engaging in consistent physical activity not only contributes to physical fitness but also plays a pivotal role in addressing the interconnected aspects of Meniere's.

1. Stress Reduction:
Regular exercise is a natural stress-reliever, aiding in the reduction of anxiety and tension—factors known to exacerbate Meniere's symptoms. Endorphins released during exercise contribute to an improved mood, fostering emotional resilience.

2. Cardiovascular Health:
Promoting cardiovascular health through regular exercise enhances blood circulation, crucial for the inner ear's function. Improved blood flow to the delicate structures implicated in Meniere's may contribute to symptom management.

3. Balance and Coordination:
Tailored exercise routines, including balance and coordination exercises, directly target the vestibular system. Strengthening these systems aids individuals in adapting to changes in equilibrium, reducing the severity and frequency of vertigo episodes.

4. Adaptability to Symptoms:
Regular exercise promotes adaptability to symptoms by enhancing overall physical conditioning. Individuals become more resilient to the challenges posed by Meniere's, fostering a proactive approach to daily living.

5. Weight Management:
Maintaining a healthy weight through regular exercise is essential for individuals with Meniere's. Excess weight can contribute to the severity of symptoms, and exercise becomes a key component in managing weight and promoting overall health.

Incorporating regular exercise into the Meniere's management toolkit is not just about physical fitness—it's a holistic approach to empowerment. By addressing stress, promoting cardiovascular health, enhancing balance, and fostering adaptability, individuals with Meniere's disease can embrace a proactive and resilient mindset as they navigate the complexities of their condition.

The Imperative of Hearing Protection

Preserving the delicate gift of hearing is a paramount concern, particularly for individuals grappling with conditions like Meniere's disease that can impact auditory function. Hearing protection becomes a crucial facet of daily life, acting as a shield against potential exacerbating factors and contributing to the overall well-being of those navigating auditory challenges.

1. Environmental Awareness:

Heightened sensitivity to sound is a common feature of Meniere's disease. Individuals are often advised to be mindful of their auditory environment, avoiding loud noises and environments that can trigger or worsen symptoms. This heightened awareness is the first line of defense in protecting the auditory apparatus.

2. Earplugs and Earmuffs:

In situations where exposure to loud noises is unavoidable, the use of earplugs or earmuffs is an effective preventative measure. Concerts, noisy workplaces, and other potentially disruptive environments can pose risks to hearing health, and these protective devices serve as guardians against auditory harm.

3. Custom Hearing Protection:

For personalized and optimal protection, custom-made earplugs molded to the individual's ear canal offer a snug fit. This tailored approach ensures both comfort and efficacy in safeguarding against excessive noise levels.

4. Noise-Canceling Headphones:

In the realm of technology, noise-canceling headphones provide a dual benefit. By reducing ambient noise, they not only offer a more serene auditory experience but also protect against potential triggers for Meniere's symptoms.

5. Limiting Exposure to Loud Devices:
Personal audio devices like headphones and earphones can contribute to hearing damage if used at high volumes for extended periods. Limiting the duration and volume of exposure to these devices is a proactive measure in maintaining auditory health.

6. Occupational Protection:
For individuals working in environments with occupational noise hazards, adherence to workplace safety guidelines and the use of protective gear, such as earmuffs or earplugs, is paramount. Employers play a vital role in providing and promoting these protective measures.

Preserving hearing health is an ongoing commitment that intertwines with the management of Meniere's disease. By embracing proactive measures such as environmental awareness, personalized protection, and adherence to safety guidelines, individuals can fortify their auditory resilience and contribute to an environment conducive to overall well-being. Hearing protection acts as a guardian, allowing individuals to navigate a world of sound with confidence and safeguarding against potential exacerbations of Meniere's symptoms.

CHAPTER FIVE

Prevention and Dietary Factors in Meniere's Management

While Meniere's disease lacks a definitive cure, a proactive approach to prevention and dietary considerations plays a pivotal role in managing symptoms and improving overall well-being. Embracing lifestyle modifications can contribute to symptom reduction and foster a sense of control in the intricate journey of Meniere's.

1. Sodium Restriction:

Dietary factors play a significant role in Meniere's management, and one key consideration is sodium restriction. High salt intake can contribute to fluid retention, potentially exacerbating inner ear symptoms.

Individuals are often advised to moderate sodium intake, reducing processed and salty foods.

2. Hydration:

Maintaining optimal hydration is crucial. Adequate water intake supports overall health and may contribute to fluid balance in the inner ear. Individuals are encouraged to stay hydrated while being mindful of their sodium levels.

3. Avoidance of Trigger Foods:

Certain foods and beverages may act as triggers for Meniere's symptoms. Caffeine, alcohol, and processed sugars are examples of potential triggers. Personalized dietary adjustments, including the identification and avoidance of trigger foods, contribute to symptom management.

4. Balanced Nutrition:

Adopting a balanced and nutrient-rich diet is essential for overall health. Incorporating a variety of fruits, vegetables, lean proteins, and whole grains provides the body with essential nutrients and supports general well-being.

5. Regular Meals and Snacks:

Maintaining regular meal patterns and incorporating healthy snacks can help stabilize blood sugar levels. Fluctuations in blood sugar can influence Meniere's symptoms, and consistent nutrition minimizes potential triggers.

6. Caffeine Moderation:

While individual responses vary, some individuals with Meniere's may find that excessive caffeine intake can exacerbate symptoms. Moderating caffeine consumption or opting for decaffeinated alternatives is a prudent dietary adjustment.

The integration of prevention strategies and mindful dietary choices empowers individuals to actively participate in their Meniere's management. A holistic approach, combining lifestyle modifications, hydration, and balanced nutrition, lays the foundation for improved symptom control and an enhanced quality of life amidst the intricacies of Meniere's disease.

Prevention Strategies for Meniere's Disease

Meniere's disease, marked by its unpredictable nature, prompts a proactive approach to symptom management and overall well-being. Prevention strategies play a pivotal role in empowering individuals to navigate the challenges posed by this intricate condition, offering a semblance of control in the face of uncertainty.

1. Environmental Awareness:

Heightened sensitivity to triggers necessitates environmental awareness. Identifying and avoiding potential triggers, such as loud noises, stressful situations, or specific foods, forms the foundation of prevention.

2. Stress Management:

Stress is a known exacerbating factor for Meniere's symptoms. Adopting stress management techniques, including mindfulness, meditation, and relaxation exercises, serves as a proactive shield against the potential impact of stress on symptom severity.

3. Regular Exercise:

Incorporating regular exercise contributes not only to physical fitness but also to overall well-being. Exercise supports cardiovascular health, aids stress reduction, and enhances adaptability to changes in balance, key components in preventing symptom escalation.

4. Dietary Modifications:

Moderating sodium intake, staying hydrated, and avoiding potential trigger foods are essential dietary prevention strategies. These measures contribute to fluid balance in the inner ear and minimize the risk of symptom exacerbation.

5. Medication Adherence:

For individuals prescribed medications to manage Meniere's symptoms, consistent adherence to the prescribed regimen is a proactive step. Medications may include diuretics to regulate fluid levels or vestibular suppressants to alleviate vertigo.

6. Regular Check-ups:

Routine medical check-ups enable healthcare professionals to monitor Meniere's progression and adjust management strategies accordingly. Regular assessments ensure timely interventions and proactive adjustments to the evolving nature of the condition.

Embracing these prevention strategies empowers individuals with Meniere's disease to actively participate in their well-being. By cultivating a proactive mindset, individuals can create a foundation for symptom control, adaptation, and an improved quality of life amidst the dynamic challenges posed by Meniere's disease.

Recognizing Early Symptoms of Meniere's Disease

Early recognition of symptoms is a pivotal aspect of managing Meniere's disease, allowing individuals to seek timely intervention and adopt strategies that mitigate the impact of the condition. Understanding the subtle cues that herald the onset of Meniere's symptoms empowers individuals to proactively navigate the complexities of this inner ear disorder.

1. Episodic Vertigo:

One of the hallmark symptoms of Meniere's disease is episodic vertigo, characterized by a sudden sensation of spinning or dizziness. Recognizing the early signs of vertigo, such as unexplained bouts of imbalance or disorientation, prompts individuals to initiate precautionary measures and seek medical evaluation.

2. Fluctuating Hearing Loss:

Meniere's often manifests as fluctuating hearing loss, typically affecting one ear. Early recognition involves being attuned to changes in hearing acuity, such as moments of muffled sounds, difficulty understanding conversations, or a sense of fullness in the ear.

3. Tinnitus:

The persistent presence of tinnitus, or ringing in the ear, is another early symptom of Meniere's disease. Recognizing the onset or exacerbation of tinnitus prompts individuals to monitor other potential symptoms and seek professional guidance.

4. Ear Fullness and Pressure:

Sensations of ear fullness or pressure are common precursors to vertigo episodes in Meniere's. Recognizing these early sensations allows individuals to implement lifestyle modifications and triggers proactive management strategies.

5. Nausea and Vomiting:

Accompanying vertigo, nausea, and vomiting are common early symptoms. Recognizing these signs facilitates prompt responses, including finding a safe environment to sit or lie down, minimizing injury risk during an episode.

6. Environmental Triggers:

Identifying potential environmental triggers, such as exposure to loud noises or stressful situations, contributes to early symptom recognition. Individuals can then proactively manage their surroundings to minimize the risk of symptom exacerbation.

Vigilance and self-awareness are essential in the early stages of Meniere's disease. Individuals who recognize these subtle but significant symptoms can collaborate with healthcare professionals to establish tailored management strategies, potentially mitigating the impact of the condition and enhancing their ability to navigate the complexities of Meniere's with resilience and foresight.

Lifestyle Changes for Preventing Meniere's Disease Symptoms

Proactive lifestyle changes stand as pivotal guardians in preventing the onset and exacerbation of Meniere's disease symptoms. Individuals navigating this intricate condition can implement tailored adjustments to their daily routines, contributing to overall well-being and minimizing the impact of triggers.

1. Dietary Modifications:
Adopting a low-sodium diet is a cornerstone of lifestyle changes for Meniere's prevention. Minimizing salt intake helps regulate fluid balance in the inner ear, reducing the risk of symptom flare-ups. Additionally, individuals may explore potential trigger foods and make personalized dietary adjustments.

2. Stress Management Techniques:
Given the intricate link between stress and Meniere's symptoms, incorporating stress management techniques becomes paramount. Practices such as meditation, deep breathing exercises, and mindfulness offer proactive tools to mitigate stressors and promote emotional well-being.

3. Regular Exercise Routine:

Engaging in a regular exercise routine contributes to overall physical health and acts as a preventive measure for Meniere's symptoms. Exercise supports cardiovascular health, aids stress reduction, and enhances adaptability to changes in balance.

4. Hydration Practices:

Maintaining optimal hydration is crucial. Adequate water intake supports fluid balance in the inner ear, potentially reducing the severity and frequency of symptoms. Consistent and mindful hydration practices contribute to overall preventive measures.

5. Environmental Awareness:

Being cognizant of environmental triggers is a proactive lifestyle change. Avoiding loud noises, managing workplace stress, and creating a calming living space contribute to a preventative environment, minimizing potential exacerbations.

By weaving these lifestyle changes into their daily fabric, individuals can proactively shape a resilient foundation against Meniere's disease symptoms. These intentional adjustments empower individuals to not merely react to the challenges of the condition but actively participate in their prevention, fostering a sense of control and well-being amidst the intricate journey of Meniere's disease.

Genetic Considerations in Meniere's Disease

While Meniere's disease is primarily considered a sporadic condition with no clear hereditary pattern, genetic factors may still play a role in predisposing individuals to this complex disorder. The intricate interplay between genetics and environmental factors remains a subject of ongoing exploration in the realm of Meniere's research.

1. Familial Clusters:
In some instances, familial clusters of Meniere's cases have been observed, suggesting a potential genetic link. However, the inheritance pattern appears complex, and multiple genetic and environmental factors likely contribute to the development of the disease.

2. Candidate Genes:
Studies have explored the role of specific genes in Meniere's disease, with a focus on those associated with inner ear function, fluid regulation, and immune response. Variations in these genes may contribute to an individual's susceptibility to the condition.

3. Multifactorial Nature:
Meniere's disease is often considered multifactorial, involving a combination of genetic and environmental elements. Individuals with a family history of the

condition may have a slightly increased risk, but the presence of specific genetic markers alone does not guarantee the development of Meniere's.

4. Research Challenges:

Unraveling the genetic tapestry of Meniere's disease poses challenges due to its complex nature and the potential influence of multiple genes. Large-scale genetic studies and advancements in genomic research are essential to gain deeper insights into the genetic components of Meniere's.

As research continues, a comprehensive understanding of the genetic considerations in Meniere's disease may offer valuable insights into its etiology, paving the way for personalized approaches to diagnosis, prevention, and management. While genetic factors contribute to the intricate puzzle of Meniere's, the interplay with environmental elements remains a critical aspect in deciphering the origins of this enigmatic condition.

CHAPTER SIX

Dietary Management in Meniere's Disease

Dietary management plays a pivotal role in the comprehensive approach to mitigating the impact of Meniere's disease, a condition characterized by inner ear disturbances. Individuals grappling with Meniere's often find relief and symptom control through strategic dietary modifications tailored to their unique needs.

1. Low-Sodium Diet:
Central to dietary management in Meniere's disease is the adoption of a low-sodium diet. Excess sodium can contribute to fluid retention in the inner ear, potentially exacerbating symptoms. Individuals are advised to limit

salt intake, avoiding processed and high-sodium foods while embracing fresh, whole foods.

2. Hydration Practices:
Maintaining optimal hydration is crucial in dietary management. Consistent and adequate water intake supports overall health and may contribute to fluid balance in the inner ear. Staying well-hydrated becomes an essential component of managing Meniere's symptoms.

3. Identification of Trigger Foods:
Understanding individual triggers is key to effective dietary management. Some individuals may find certain foods or beverages, such as caffeine, alcohol, or specific additives, act as triggers for their symptoms. Identifying and avoiding these trigger foods enhances symptom control.

4. Balanced Nutrition:
Embracing a balanced and nutrient-rich diet contributes to overall well-being. Incorporating a variety of fruits, vegetables, lean proteins, and whole grains provides essential nutrients that support the body's resilience and adaptability.

5. Caffeine Moderation:
While individual responses vary, moderation of caffeine intake is often recommended in dietary management.

Some individuals with Meniere's may find that excessive caffeine consumption can exacerbate symptoms, and adjusting intake levels becomes a proactive measure.

6. Individualized Approaches:
Dietary management in Meniere's is inherently individualized. Recognizing that responses to specific foods and dietary patterns vary, individuals often work with healthcare professionals or registered dietitians to tailor dietary strategies to their unique needs and preferences.

By actively engaging in dietary management, individuals with Meniere's disease can empower themselves in the quest for symptom control and improved quality of life. This approach, complemented by lifestyle modifications and medical interventions, contributes to a holistic framework that addresses the multifaceted nature of Meniere's, fostering wellness and resilience in the face of this intricate condition.

The Crucial Role of Salt Intake in Meniere's Disease

Salt intake stands at the forefront of dietary considerations for individuals grappling with Meniere's disease. The delicate equilibrium within the inner ear is profoundly influenced by sodium levels, making strategic salt management a cornerstone in the comprehensive approach to symptom control.

1. Fluid Regulation in the Inner Ear:
Excess sodium in the body can disrupt fluid balance, leading to fluid retention in the inner ear. For individuals with Meniere's disease, this fluid imbalance can contribute to the severity and frequency of symptoms, including vertigo, hearing loss, and tinnitus.

2. Low-Sodium Diet:
Adopting a low-sodium diet is a primary recommendation in Meniere's dietary management. This involves reducing salt intake by avoiding high-sodium processed foods, canned goods, and salty snacks. Fresh, whole foods and culinary herbs become valuable allies in enhancing flavor without relying on excess salt.

3. Minimizing Fluid Retention:
Strategic salt management aims to minimize fluid retention, thereby alleviating the pressure within the delicate structures of the inner ear. This proactive approach supports individuals in regaining control over their symptoms and enhances overall well-being.

4. Individualized Approaches:

Recognizing that salt sensitivity varies among individuals, a one-size-fits-all approach may not suffice. Personalized dietary consultations with healthcare professionals or registered dietitians enable individuals to tailor salt intake to their unique needs, considering factors such as age, overall health, and lifestyle.

In the intricate dance of Meniere's disease, where the slightest imbalance can trigger disruptive symptoms, understanding and managing salt intake become integral steps in the journey towards wellness. By embracing a low-sodium lifestyle, individuals empower themselves with a potent tool to navigate the complexities of Meniere's, fostering a sense of control and equilibrium in their daily lives.

The Impact of Hydration in Meniere's Disease

Hydration emerges as a vital player in the symphony of strategies for managing Meniere's disease, an intricate condition affecting the inner ear. Optimal fluid balance is crucial for inner ear health, and strategic hydration practices become a key component in alleviating symptoms and fostering overall well-being.

1. Fluid Balance in the Inner Ear:

The inner ear, responsible for auditory and vestibular functions, relies on delicate fluid balance. Adequate hydration supports the stability of this fluid environment, potentially reducing the severity and frequency of Meniere's symptoms such as vertigo, hearing loss, and tinnitus.

2. Prevention of Dehydration:

Dehydration can exacerbate Meniere's symptoms. Maintaining proper hydration levels is essential to prevent the concentration of salts and minerals in the body, which can impact the fluid composition in the inner ear.

3. Enhancing Adaptability:

Hydration contributes to the body's adaptability to changes in fluid dynamics. Individuals with Meniere's are encouraged to stay consistently hydrated, supporting their ability to adapt to triggers and changes in their environment.

4. Holistic Well-Being:

Beyond its specific impact on Meniere's symptoms, hydration is foundational to overall health and well-being. Proper fluid intake supports cardiovascular health, aids digestion, and contributes to cognitive function—elements that collectively enhance the resilience of individuals managing Meniere's disease.

As individuals navigate the labyrinthine challenges of Meniere's, acknowledging the profound impact of hydration on inner ear health becomes a proactive step. By incorporating mindful hydration practices into their daily routines, individuals empower themselves with a fundamental tool to support the delicate balance within the inner ear, fostering a sense of equilibrium amidst the complexities of Meniere's disease.

A Dietary Guide for Meniere's Symptom Management

Diet plays a pivotal role in the management of Meniere's disease, with strategic choices influencing symptom severity and overall well-being. Understanding which foods to include and avoid empowers individuals to craft a personalized menu that supports inner ear health and minimizes potential triggers.

Foods to Include:

1. Fresh Fruits and Vegetables:
   A rainbow of fruits and vegetables provides essential vitamins, minerals, and antioxidants. These nutrient-rich choices contribute to overall well-being and support the body's resilience.

2. Lean Proteins:

Incorporating lean protein sources such as poultry, fish, tofu, and legumes offers essential amino acids without excess saturated fats. Protein is crucial for muscle health and overall energy.

3. Whole Grains:

Opting for whole grains like brown rice, quinoa, and oats provides fiber and sustained energy. These grains contribute to balanced nutrition and support digestive health.

4. Nuts and Seeds:

Rich in healthy fats, nuts and seeds are valuable additions. Omega-3 fatty acids found in certain nuts and seeds may have anti-inflammatory properties beneficial for individuals with Meniere's.

5. Water and Herbal Teas:

Adequate hydration is fundamental. Water and herbal teas support fluid balance in the body, contributing to inner ear health. Limiting caffeine intake, found in some teas, is advisable for those sensitive to its effects.

Foods to Avoid:

1. High-Sodium Foods:

Sodium is a primary concern for individuals with Meniere's. Processed foods, canned goods, and salty snacks should be minimized to reduce the risk of fluid retention in the inner ear.

2. Caffeine and Stimulants:

Excessive caffeine intake may exacerbate Meniere's symptoms. Monitoring and moderating caffeine consumption, found in coffee, tea, and some sodas, is prudent.

3. Alcohol:

Alcohol can impact fluid balance and trigger symptoms in some individuals. Limiting alcohol intake or avoiding it altogether is recommended.

4. Processed and Trigger Foods:

Identification and avoidance of trigger foods vary among individuals. Common triggers include processed sugars, certain additives, and foods that individuals have personally identified as problematic.

Crafting a Meniere's-friendly menu involves thoughtful consideration of individual sensitivities and preferences. Consulting with healthcare professionals, including dietitians, supports the creation of a personalized dietary plan that aligns with overall health goals and minimizes the impact of Meniere's symptoms.

Supplements and Potential Benefits for Meniere's Disease

In the intricate journey of managing Meniere's disease, strategic supplementation can be a valuable ally, offering potential benefits in supporting overall health and mitigating the impact of symptoms. While individual responses vary, certain supplements have been explored for their potential positive effects on Meniere's-related challenges.

1. Vitamin B12:

Vitamin B12 plays a crucial role in nerve function and may have implications for individuals with Meniere's disease, particularly those with documented deficiencies. Adequate B12 levels contribute to overall neurological health and may support the nervous system.

2. Magnesium:

Magnesium, known for its role in muscle and nerve function, has been studied for its potential benefits in managing Meniere's symptoms. Some individuals report symptom relief with magnesium supplementation, emphasizing the importance of personalized approaches.

3. Omega-3 Fatty Acids:

Found in fish oil supplements, omega-3 fatty acids possess anti-inflammatory properties. While research on omega-3 supplementation for Meniere's is limited, some individuals incorporate fish oil for its potential positive impact on inflammation and overall cardiovascular health.

4. Vitamin D:

Vitamin D, vital for bone health and immune function, has garnered attention in Meniere's research. While studies are ongoing, maintaining optimal vitamin D levels may contribute to general well-being for individuals managing Meniere's.

5. Ginkgo Biloba:

Ginkgo biloba, an herbal supplement, has been explored for its potential benefits in supporting inner ear circulation. Some individuals report improvements in tinnitus and vertigo symptoms with ginkgo biloba supplementation, though individual responses vary.

6. Coenzyme Q10 (CoQ10):

CoQ10, an antioxidant involved in cellular energy production, has been considered for its potential benefits in supporting mitochondrial function. Some individuals find CoQ10 supplementation beneficial in managing fatigue and promoting overall energy levels.

Before incorporating supplements, consultation with healthcare professionals is crucial to ensure personalized and safe approaches. Dosages, potential interactions with medications, and individual health profiles should be considered. Additionally, the holistic integration of supplements into a comprehensive approach, including dietary modifications and lifestyle changes, enhances their potential benefits in navigating the complexities of Meniere's disease.

CHAPTER SEVEN

Symptom Management in

Meniere's Disease

Symptom management stands as a pivotal aspect of the comprehensive approach to Meniere's disease, aiming to alleviate the disruptive impact of vertigo, hearing loss, tinnitus, and ear fullness. Individuals navigating the complex landscape of Meniere's employ a multifaceted toolkit to proactively address and mitigate these challenging symptoms.

1. Vestibular Rehabilitation Exercises:
  Tailored exercises designed to improve balance and coordination, known as vestibular rehabilitation, are key components of managing vertigo. These exercises enhance the brain's ability to adapt to changes in the

inner ear, reducing the severity and frequency of vertigo episodes.

2. Medications:

Medications may be prescribed to manage specific symptoms. Diuretics help regulate fluid balance, reducing inner ear pressure, while vestibular suppressants alleviate vertigo symptoms. Individual responses vary, and medication management is personalized based on the specific needs of each individual.

3. Hearing Aids:

For those experiencing hearing loss, hearing aids are valuable tools that enhance auditory input. Customized to individual hearing needs, hearing aids contribute to improved communication and overall quality of life.

4. Tinnitus Management Strategies:

Tinnitus, or ringing in the ears, is addressed through various management strategies. Sound therapy, cognitive-behavioral therapy, and relaxation techniques can help individuals habituate to or cope with tinnitus, minimizing its impact on daily life.

5. Lifestyle Modifications:

Implementing lifestyle changes, including dietary modifications, stress management, and hydration practices, contributes to overall symptom control.

Individuals often find that a holistic approach that encompasses multiple facets of their daily lives enhances their ability to manage Meniere's symptoms effectively.

By weaving these strategies into a cohesive and individualized management plan, individuals with Meniere's disease harmonize their wellness journey. Symptom management is not a one-size-fits-all endeavor, but a dynamic interplay of strategies that empowers individuals to navigate the intricacies of Meniere's with resilience and adaptability. Regular communication with healthcare professionals ensures ongoing adjustments to the management plan, creating a roadmap for sustained well-being amidst the challenges posed by Meniere's disease.

Overview of Medications in Meniere's Disease Management

Medications play a crucial role in managing the symptoms of Meniere's disease, a condition characterized by inner ear disturbances leading to vertigo, hearing loss, tinnitus, and ear fullness. While there is no cure for Meniere's, medications are employed to alleviate symptoms and enhance overall quality of life for individuals navigating this intricate disorder.

1. Diuretics:

Diuretics, such as hydrochlorothiazide or triamterene, are commonly prescribed to regulate fluid balance in the body. By reducing excess fluid, particularly in the inner ear, diuretics aim to minimize the frequency and severity of vertigo episodes associated with Meniere's.

2. Vestibular Suppressants:

Medications like meclizine or diazepam act as vestibular suppressants, targeting the vestibular system to alleviate symptoms of vertigo. While these medications do not address the root cause of Meniere's, they provide relief during acute episodes and enhance overall comfort.

3. Anti-nausea Medications:

Nausea and vomiting often accompany vertigo episodes. Medications like ondansetron or promethazine may be prescribed to manage these symptoms, providing individuals with a more tolerable experience during vertiginous episodes.

4. Corticosteroids:

Corticosteroids, such as prednisone, may be utilized to reduce inflammation in the inner ear. While their use is typically short-term due to potential side effects, corticosteroids can be beneficial in certain cases to alleviate symptoms and promote recovery.

5. Betahistine:

Betahistine is a medication that may improve blood flow in the inner ear. While its effectiveness is debated, some individuals find relief from symptoms such as vertigo and tinnitus with betahistine supplementation.

6. Anti-anxiety Medications:

Managing the emotional impact of Meniere's is essential. Anti-anxiety medications, such as benzodiazepines, may be prescribed to individuals experiencing heightened anxiety or stress related to their symptoms.

It's crucial for individuals with Meniere's to work closely with healthcare professionals to determine the most suitable medication regimen based on their specific symptoms and overall health. Medication management is often part of a comprehensive approach that includes lifestyle modifications, dietary adjustments, and other strategies to enhance overall well-being amidst the challenges of Meniere's disease. Regular communication with healthcare providers allows for ongoing evaluation and adjustments to ensure optimal symptom relief.

Benefits and Side Effects of Medications in Meniere's Disease Management

In the intricate landscape of Meniere's disease management, medications serve as both allies and potential challengers. Understanding the benefits and potential side effects of these medications is essential for individuals navigating this complex condition, aiming for symptom relief while minimizing unwanted consequences.

Benefits:

1. Symptom Relief:
The primary benefit of medications in Meniere's disease management is symptom relief. Whether targeting vertigo, nausea, or anxiety associated with Meniere's symptoms, medications aim to enhance overall comfort and quality of life for individuals grappling with this inner ear disorder.

2. Improved Functionality:
By addressing symptoms such as vertigo and hearing loss, medications contribute to improved functionality. Individuals can experience enhanced daily living, communication, and emotional well-being, fostering a

sense of normalcy amidst the challenges posed by Meniere's.

3. Enhanced Quality of Life:

Medications play a crucial role in enhancing the overall quality of life for individuals with Meniere's. Through symptom management, individuals can engage more fully in work, social activities, and relationships, mitigating the impact of Meniere's on their daily experiences.

Side Effects:

1. Sedation and Drowsiness:

Some medications used to manage Meniere's symptoms, such as vestibular suppressants or anti-anxiety medications, may cause sedation and drowsiness. Finding the right balance to alleviate symptoms without causing excessive drowsiness is a delicate consideration.

2. Gastrointestinal Distress:

Diuretics, commonly prescribed for fluid regulation, can lead to increased urination and potential gastrointestinal distress. Individuals may experience dehydration or electrolyte imbalances, necessitating close monitoring by healthcare professionals.

3. Corticosteroid Side Effects:

While corticosteroids can reduce inflammation in the inner ear, their long-term use may lead to various side effects, including weight gain, mood changes, and increased susceptibility to infections.

4. Dependency and Tolerance:

Some medications, particularly anti-anxiety medications or pain relievers, carry the risk of dependency and tolerance. Careful management and communication with healthcare providers are essential to prevent unintended consequences of long-term medication use.

Navigating the benefits and side effects of medications in Meniere's disease involves an ongoing dialogue between individuals and their healthcare providers. Balancing the positive impact on symptoms with potential challenges requires personalized approaches, emphasizing the importance of open communication, regular check-ups, and collaborative decision-making. As the landscape of Meniere's management evolves, ongoing research and advancements offer hope for even more effective and tailored approaches to alleviate symptoms and enhance the well-being of those living with this intricate condition.

CHAPTER EIGHT

Surgical and Invasive Options in

Meniere's Disease

For individuals grappling with severe and unresponsive Meniere's disease symptoms, surgical and invasive interventions may be considered as a last resort. These options aim to address the root causes of Meniere's and provide a more enduring solution to the challenges posed by this complex inner ear disorder.

1. Endolymphatic Sac Decompression Surgery:
   This surgical procedure involves creating a small incision behind the ear to access the endolymphatic sac—a structure believed to play a role in fluid regulation in the inner ear. Decompression aims to

improve fluid drainage and reduce the frequency and severity of vertigo episodes.

2. Vestibular Nerve Section (Vestibular Neurectomy):
Vestibular nerve section involves surgically disconnecting the vestibular nerve, which carries signals related to balance and spatial orientation. By interrupting these signals, vestibular nerve section aims to alleviate vertigo symptoms.

3. Labyrinthectomy:
In cases of profound hearing loss and debilitating vertigo, labyrinthectomy may be considered. This invasive procedure involves removing the entire inner ear, including the cochlea and vestibular system, to eliminate both hearing and balance function on the affected side.

4. Cochlear Implantation:
For individuals with severe hearing loss in the affected ear, cochlear implantation may be an option. Cochlear implants are electronic devices that stimulate the auditory nerve, providing a sense of sound to individuals with significant hearing impairment.

5. Intratympanic Gentamicin Therapy:
This minimally invasive procedure involves injecting the antibiotic gentamicin into the middle ear to selectively damage the inner ear structures responsible

for vertigo. While effective in reducing vertigo, this approach carries potential risks, including hearing loss.

6. Hydroxychloroquine Treatment:
   Experimental treatments, such as the use of hydroxychloroquine, are being explored to modulate the immune response and potentially reduce symptoms in some individuals with Meniere's.

While surgical and invasive options offer potential relief for some individuals, these interventions come with risks and considerations. Consultation with a multidisciplinary team, including ear specialists and surgeons, is essential to determine the most appropriate approach based on an individual's specific symptoms, overall health, and treatment goals. The decision to pursue surgical or invasive options in Meniere's disease is highly individualized and involves careful consideration of the potential benefits and risks associated with each intervention.

When Surgery May be Considered in Meniere's Disease

Surgery emerges as a contemplative option in the journey of Meniere's disease when conservative approaches and medical interventions prove insufficient in managing debilitating symptoms. The decision to explore surgical options is nuanced, considering the severity of symptoms, their impact on daily life, and the individual's responsiveness to other treatments.

1. Persistent and Severe Vertigo:

Surgery may be considered when vertigo remains persistent and severe, significantly affecting an individual's quality of life. Despite medication and lifestyle modifications, if vertigo episodes persist and compromise daily functioning, surgical intervention becomes a potential avenue for relief.

2. Unresponsive to Medications:

If medications fail to adequately control symptoms or if individuals experience intolerable side effects, surgical options may be explored. The goal is to address the root causes of Meniere's disease and offer a more enduring solution.

3. Progressive Hearing Loss:

When Meniere's disease leads to progressive hearing loss, and hearing aids or other interventions are no longer sufficient, surgical options like cochlear implantation or labyrinthectomy may be considered to address both hearing and balance issues.

4. Deteriorating Quality of Life:

Surgical considerations extend beyond the physical symptoms to encompass the overall impact on an individual's well-being. If Meniere's significantly compromises one's ability to work, engage in social activities, or maintain emotional well-being, surgery may be explored to improve the overall quality of life.

5. Failure of Conservative Measures:

When conservative measures, such as dietary modifications, lifestyle changes, and medical treatments, prove ineffective in managing symptoms, surgical options become a strategic pathway. The decision is often made collaboratively between the individual and their healthcare team after thorough evaluation and discussion of potential benefits and risks.

6. Balancing Risks and Benefits:

Surgical considerations involve a careful evaluation of potential risks and benefits. Factors such as age, overall health, and individual treatment goals play a crucial role in determining the appropriateness of surgical interventions.

As Meniere's disease manifests uniquely in each individual, the decision to pursue surgery is highly personalized. A comprehensive evaluation by a team of specialists, including ear, nose, and throat (ENT) surgeons, audiologists, and other healthcare professionals, is crucial to ensure that surgical options align with the specific needs and circumstances of the individual. Open communication, thorough evaluation, and collaborative decision-making contribute to a well-informed and empowered approach when contemplating surgery in the management of Meniere's disease.

Risks and Benefits of Surgical Interventions in Meniere's Disease

Surgical interventions in Meniere's disease are considered when conservative measures and medical treatments fall short in providing relief from debilitating symptoms. Understanding the potential risks and benefits associated with these procedures is crucial for individuals contemplating surgery as a strategic step in managing this intricate inner ear disorder.

Benefits:

1. Vertigo Relief:
One of the primary benefits of surgical interventions is the potential for significant vertigo relief. Procedures such as vestibular nerve section or endolymphatic sac decompression aim to address the underlying causes of

vertigo, providing individuals with a reprieve from the intense and unpredictable episodes.

2. Hearing Improvement:
Certain surgical options, like cochlear implantation, may offer the possibility of hearing improvement for individuals experiencing profound hearing loss. While not a guaranteed outcome, cochlear implants provide a technological solution to enhance auditory function.

3. Enhanced Quality of Life:
Successfully managing Meniere's symptoms through surgery can contribute to an enhanced overall quality of life. Improved functionality, reduced symptom severity, and the potential for a return to daily activities with greater ease are significant advantages for individuals navigating Meniere's.

Risks:

1. Hearing Loss:
Surgical interventions, especially those involving the inner ear, carry the risk of hearing loss. Procedures like labyrinthectomy or vestibular nerve section may result in a sacrifice of hearing function to achieve vertigo relief.

2. Balance Issues:
While the goal of surgery is often to address imbalance, certain procedures can potentially lead to persistent or

new balance issues. The delicate equilibrium of the inner ear is intricately connected, and surgical interventions may disrupt this balance.

3. Infection and Complications:

As with any surgery, the risk of infection and other complications exists. Invasive procedures, such as labyrinthectomy, necessitate careful post-operative monitoring to minimize the risk of infections that could impact recovery.

4. Individual Variability:

Responses to surgical interventions vary widely among individuals. What works well for one person may not yield the same outcomes for another. Individual factors, including overall health and responsiveness to surgery, contribute to the variability in outcomes.

When contemplating surgical interventions for Meniere's disease, a collaborative approach involving thorough discussions with healthcare professionals is crucial. Detailed consultations with ear, nose, and throat (ENT) specialists and a comprehensive understanding of individual health profiles contribute to informed decision-making. Ultimately, the balance between the potential benefits and risks is unique to each individual, and the decision to pursue surgical intervention should align with the individual's treatment goals, preferences, and overall well-being.

CHAPTER NINE

Real-Life Experiences with

Meniere's Disease

Behind the clinical descriptions and medical interventions lies a tapestry of real-life experiences woven by individuals confronting the challenges of Meniere's disease. These narratives, diverse and dynamic, offer insights into the profound impact of this inner ear disorder on daily life and the strategies employed to navigate its complexities.

1. The Unpredictability of Vertigo:
   Many individuals with Meniere's share a common thread—the unpredictable nature of vertigo attacks. These episodes, often accompanied by nausea and a sense of disorientation, can strike at any moment,

disrupting routines and instilling a constant vigilance that shapes their daily lives.

2. Navigating Hearing Loss:

Hearing loss, a hallmark of Meniere's, transforms communication dynamics. Real-life experiences often revolve around adapting to changes in social interactions, employment, and personal relationships. Hearing aids, cochlear implants, and assistive technologies become integral tools in this journey.

3. Coping with Tinnitus:

The persistent presence of tinnitus, or ringing in the ears, is a shared reality. Real-life narratives reveal a spectrum of coping strategies, from incorporating white noise to mindfulness techniques, each individual crafting a unique approach to minimize the impact of this auditory companion.

4. Strategies for Daily Living:

Everyday activities take on new dimensions for individuals with Meniere's. Grocery shopping, navigating crowded spaces, or even enjoying a leisurely walk become strategic endeavors as they consider triggers and potential challenges.

5. Balancing Emotional Well-Being:

Emotional resilience is a common theme in real-life experiences. The emotional toll of Meniere's, including anxiety and frustration, is palpable. Individuals share stories of seeking support, whether through counseling, support groups, or connecting with others who understand the intricacies of their journey.

6. Hope and Adaptability:
Amidst the challenges, real-life narratives are imbued with hope and adaptability. Individuals share stories of finding effective treatments, developing personalized coping mechanisms, and embracing a mindset that prioritizes well-being.

In these real-life experiences, a mosaic of strength, adaptability, and community emerges. Each individual's journey is a testament to resilience, as they navigate the ebbs and flows of Meniere's disease with courage and determination. Through these narratives, a supportive community emerges, offering solace and inspiration to those at various stages of their Meniere's journey.

Effective Strategies Shared by Individuals with Meniere's Disease

Amidst the complexities of Meniere's disease, individuals share a tapestry of strategies that have become guiding stars in their journey. These personal anecdotes illuminate the resilience and resourcefulness of those grappling with the challenges of vertigo, hearing loss, and tinnitus.

1. Mindful Triggers Management:

Many individuals highlight the effectiveness of identifying and managing triggers. From dietary modifications to stress reduction techniques, adopting a mindful approach to potential triggers forms a cornerstone in their strategies.

2. Embracing Hearing Technologies:

Personal stories often underscore the transformative power of hearing aids and cochlear implants. Embracing these technologies not only improves communication but also enhances overall quality of life, enabling individuals to stay connected with their surroundings.

3. Creating Safe Spaces:

Strategic adaptations in daily living, such as organizing home environments for safety and minimizing potential hazards, have proven effective. Creating safe spaces becomes a tangible way to mitigate the impact of unexpected vertigo episodes.

4. Soundscapes and White Noise:

Taming the persistent symphony of tinnitus often involves crafting personalized soundscapes. From white noise machines to calming music, individuals share how these auditory allies help mask the ringing in their ears and promote a sense of tranquility.

5. Cultivating Emotional Well-being:
  Personal stories emphasize the importance of cultivating emotional resilience. Engaging in activities that bring joy, seeking counseling, and connecting with support groups contribute to a robust emotional well-being that empowers individuals to navigate the emotional roller coaster of Meniere's.

These shared strategies not only reflect the diverse approaches individuals employ but also highlight the adaptive spirit inherent in those living with Meniere's disease. The collective wisdom drawn from these strategies serves as a beacon of hope, offering insights and inspiration to others on similar journeys, fostering a sense of empowerment in the face of a condition that demands ongoing adaptation and resilience.

Overcoming Challenges in the Meniere's Journey

Individuals living with Meniere's disease embody resilience as they navigate a labyrinth of challenges, each triumph contributing to a narrative of strength and adaptation. From the tumultuous waves of vertigo to the strains of hearing loss and persistent tinnitus, these stories reflect the triumphs that emerge amidst the complexities of Meniere's.

1. Navigating Unpredictable Vertigo:

Overcoming the unpredictability of vertigo stands as a significant triumph. Individuals share stories of learning to manage and adapt to sudden bouts of dizziness, implementing strategies to mitigate their impact on daily activities, and cultivating resilience in the face of uncertainty.

2. Adapting to Hearing Loss:

The challenge of hearing loss transforms into triumph through adaptation. Stories abound of individuals embracing hearing aids, cochlear implants, and assistive technologies, fostering not only improved communication but also a renewed sense of connection with the world around them.

3. Conquering Tinnitus Dissonance:

Overcoming the persistent symphony of tinnitus becomes a triumph of the mind. Personal stories resonate with strategies that tame the ringing in the ears, allowing individuals to reclaim moments of quietude and find solace amidst the auditory chaos.

4. Thriving Despite Emotional Impact:

Triumph over the emotional impact of Meniere's disease is a common thread. Individuals share their journey towards emotional well-being, conquering anxiety, stress, and the emotional toll of living with a chronic condition, and finding resilience in fostering mental health.

As these personal narratives unfold, a collective tale of triumph emerges—a testament to the indomitable spirit of those facing the challenges of Meniere's disease. Through each conquered obstacle, individuals not only find strength within themselves but also offer inspiration and hope to others embarking on similar journeys.

CHAPTER TEN

Living a Fulfilling Life with

Meniere's Disease

Living with Meniere's disease presents unique challenges, but countless individuals carve pathways to fulfillment, resilience, and joy despite the intricacies of this inner ear disorder. By embracing adaptive strategies and cultivating a holistic approach to well-being, many find that a fulfilling life is not only attainable but can thrive amidst the complexities of Meniere's.

1. Adaptive Strategies:
   Individuals living with Meniere's often discover a repertoire of adaptive strategies that allow them to engage fully in life. From mindful trigger management to strategic planning for unpredictable vertigo episodes,

these adaptive approaches form the foundation for a fulfilling daily existence.

2. Holistic Wellness:

Fostering overall well-being becomes a cornerstone for a fulfilling life. Integrating physical, emotional, and mental wellness through activities such as regular exercise, stress management, and mindfulness practices contributes to a balanced and resilient lifestyle.

3. Navigating Social Interactions:

Despite challenges like hearing loss, individuals cultivate meaningful connections by effectively navigating social interactions. Communication tools, assistive devices, and open communication with others play pivotal roles in maintaining vibrant relationships and social engagement.

4. Pursuing Passions:

Many individuals with Meniere's disease find fulfillment in pursuing their passions. Whether through creative outlets, hobbies, or activities that bring joy, investing time and energy into personal interests becomes a powerful source of fulfillment and purpose.

5. Seeking Professional Support:

Engaging with healthcare professionals, including ear specialists, therapists, and support groups, enhances the journey towards fulfillment. Seeking professional guidance fosters a sense of empowerment, providing valuable tools and insights for managing both the physical and emotional aspects of Meniere's.

6. Community Connection:

The sense of community becomes a vital component of a fulfilling life. Connecting with others who share similar experiences fosters understanding, empathy, and a shared resilience that transforms the Meniere's journey into a collective and supportive endeavor.

By weaving together adaptive strategies, holistic wellness practices, and a community-focused mindset, individuals with Meniere's disease forge a path to a fulfilling life. While challenges persist, the triumphs, connections, and moments of joy become the threads that contribute to a rich and vibrant tapestry of living with resilience and purpose despite the complexities of Meniere's.

Key Takeaways

Understanding Meniere's disease involves delving into its intricacies, from vertigo to hearing loss and the emotional toll it exacts. Through this exploration, key takeaways emerge to guide individuals on their journey:

1. Individualized Journey:
   Meniere's manifests uniquely in each person, emphasizing the need for an individualized approach to management. What works for one may not be universal, necessitating personalized strategies and solutions.

2. Holistic Well-being:
   A holistic approach to well-being proves pivotal. Managing Meniere's extends beyond symptom control to encompass physical, emotional, and social aspects. Strategies like exercise, stress management, and community connection contribute to a balanced and resilient life.

3. Adaptive Strategies:
   Navigating the unpredictability of Meniere's demands adaptive strategies. From mindful triggers management to embracing assistive devices, individuals discover a toolkit of techniques that empower them to lead fulfilling lives despite the challenges.

4. Community Support:
   The strength of community support shines through. Engaging with healthcare professionals, connecting with support groups, and sharing personal stories create a sense of solidarity and understanding, fostering a supportive ecosystem.

5. Resilience and Triumph:

Personal narratives underscore the resilience inherent in those living with Meniere's. Triumphs over vertigo, hearing loss, and emotional challenges weave a tapestry of strength, offering inspiration and hope for others on similar journeys.

In summary, Meniere's disease, while intricate, can be navigated with a tailored and holistic approach, adaptive strategies, and the collective strength of a supportive community. Living a fulfilling life with Meniere's involves embracing resilience, pursuing passions, and finding joy amidst the challenges, creating a narrative of triumph and empowerment.

Nurturing Hope for Meniere's Warriors

For those navigating the labyrinth of Meniere's disease, every step may feel like a triumph. In the midst of vertigo's unpredictability, the persistence of tinnitus, and the adjustment to hearing loss, it's essential to recognize the strength within and embrace a spirit of encouragement.

1. Your Journey, Your Pace:

Meniere's is a deeply personal journey, and there is no predetermined timeline for mastery. Embrace your unique path, acknowledging that healing and adaptation occur at your own pace.

2. Celebrate Small Victories:

Amidst the challenges, celebrate the small victories. Whether it's a day free from vertigo, a moment of clarity in communication, or a successful adaptation strategy, these triumphs illuminate the resilience within you.

3. Connect with Community:

You are not alone. Connect with the vibrant Meniere's community—share your experiences, glean insights from others, and draw strength from the collective wisdom that emerges when stories intertwine.

4. Seek Professional Support:

Reach out to healthcare professionals who specialize in Meniere's disease. Their expertise and guidance can provide valuable tools, strategies, and a comprehensive approach to managing the various facets of the condition.

5. Embrace Adaptability:

Adaptability is your superpower. Explore adaptive strategies for daily living, discover technologies that enhance communication, and find comfort in the flexibility that allows you to navigate the ebb and flow of Meniere's.

In the intricate tapestry of Meniere's, your resilience is the thread that binds every challenge and triumph. Let encouragement be your companion, nurturing hope, and reminding you that, despite the complexities, a fulfilling and joyful life is both achievable and well-deserved.

The Vital Role of Ongoing Medical Care and Adaptation in Meniere's Journey

In the labyrinth of Meniere's disease, the significance of ongoing medical care and adaptation cannot be overstated. Regular medical check-ups serve as compass points, guiding individuals through the twists and turns of their unique Meniere's journey.

1. Dynamic Nature of Meniere's:
   Meniere's is a dynamic condition, evolving over time. Ongoing medical care ensures that healthcare professionals can assess changes, fine-tune treatment plans, and offer timely interventions, adapting to the ever-changing landscape of symptoms.

2. Holistic Well-being:

Regular medical care extends beyond symptom management, encompassing holistic well-being. Monitoring not only the physical aspects of Meniere's but also the emotional and social dimensions ensures a comprehensive approach that nurtures overall health.

3. Adaptation Strategies:

The adaptation is a constant ally. Regular check-ups provide opportunities to explore and refine adaptive strategies. From lifestyle modifications to incorporating new technologies, these adaptations empower individuals to navigate daily life with resilience.

4. Preventing Complications:

Timely medical care plays a preventive role, addressing potential complications. Monitoring hearing health, managing triggers, and addressing emerging issues head-on contribute to preventing the exacerbation of symptoms and improving long-term outcomes.

5. Empowerment Through Knowledge:

Ongoing medical care empowers individuals with knowledge. Understanding the nuances of Meniere's and staying informed about emerging treatments, research, and community resources equips individuals to make informed decisions and actively participate in their healthcare journey.

In the symphony of Meniere's, ongoing medical care and adaptation are the conductor's baton, orchestrating a harmonious and resilient life. Regular check-ups not only monitor the intricacies of the condition but also serve as waypoints for individuals, guiding them towards a future filled with adaptive strategies, informed decisions, and sustained well-being.